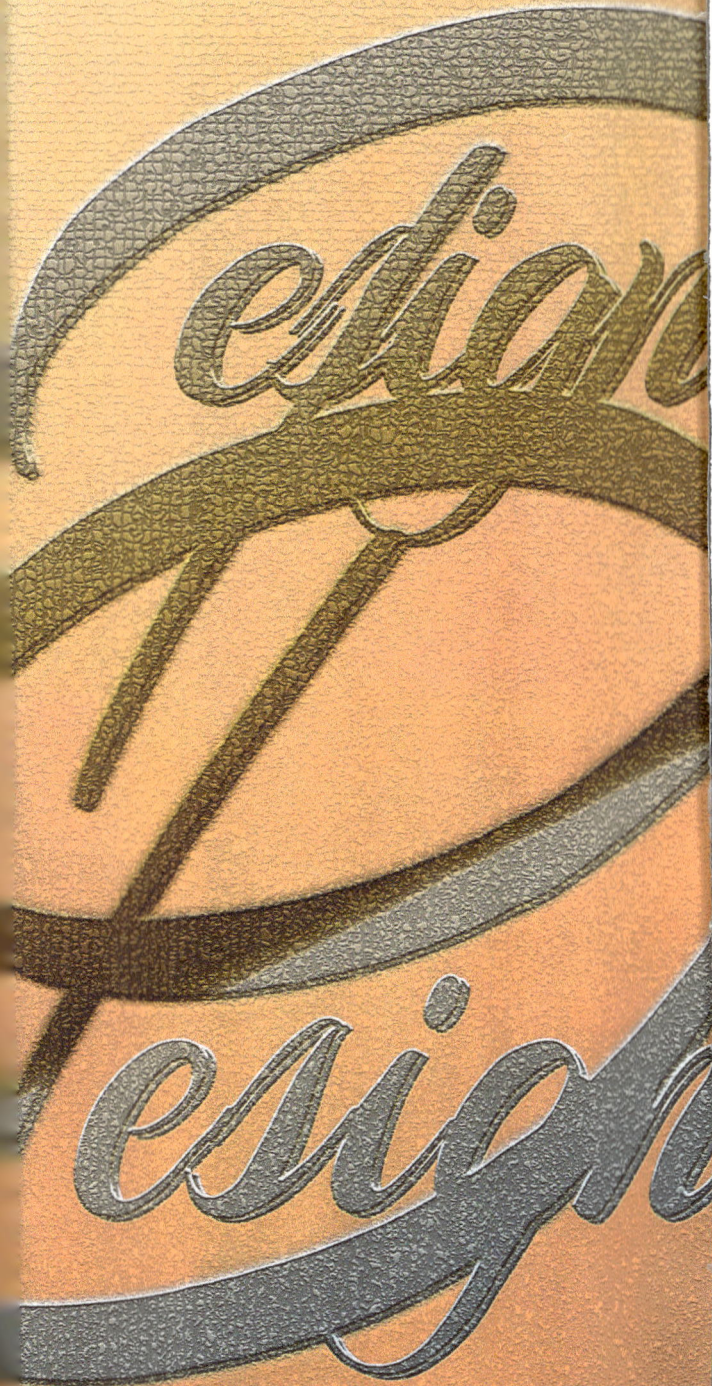

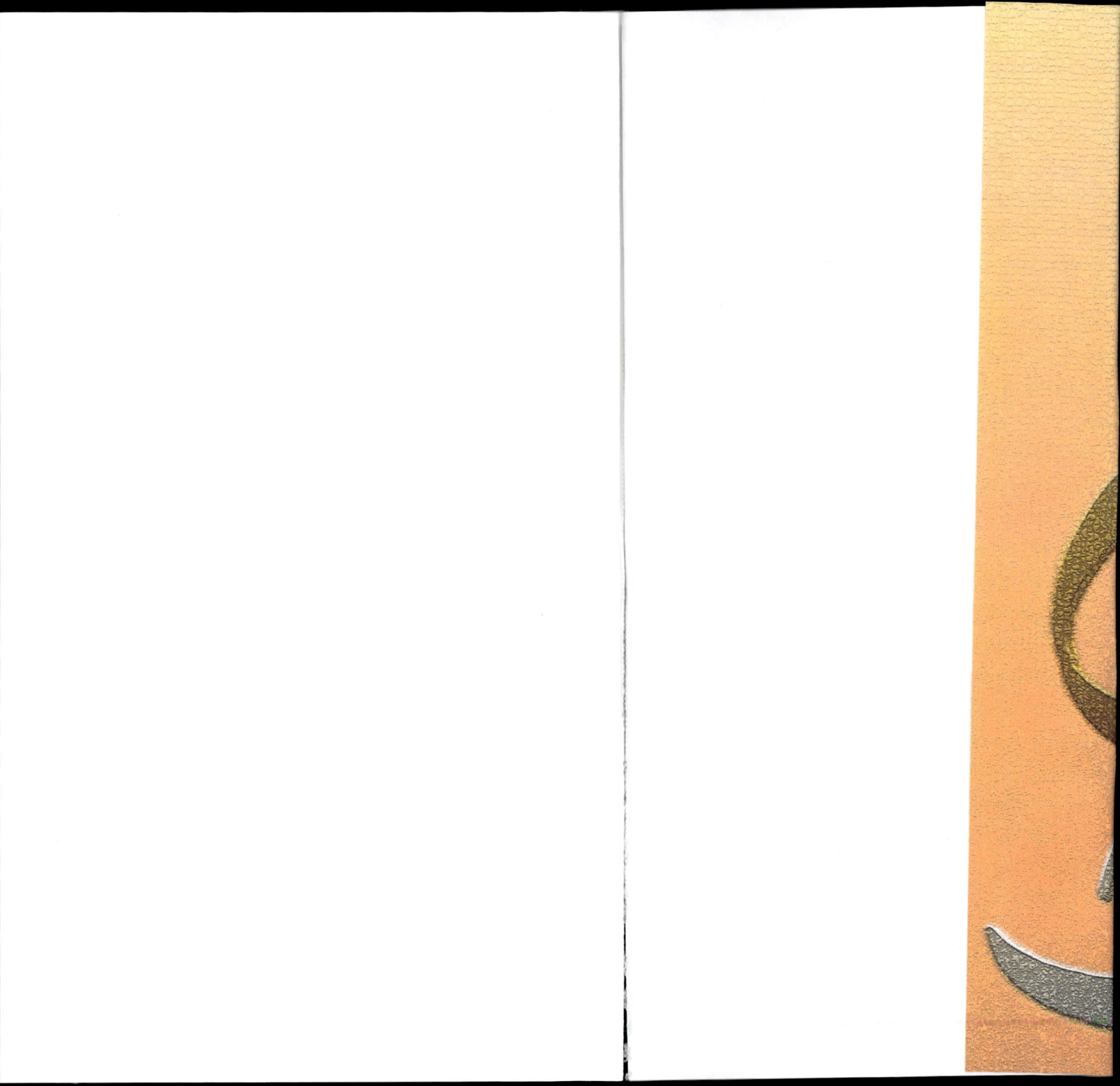

alking?

Oh yes!

Sense?

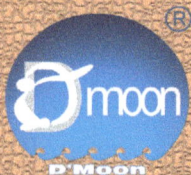

Credit goes to
author Astron Hues,
and the team of designers,
photographers, cartoonists,
and editors at the publisher: D'Moon

ISBN: 978-1-933187-14-3

Slight variations may occur
as part of the print-on-demand process
since each book is manufactured in its entirety.

Your feedback is most welcome ~
publisher@worldculturepictorial.com

Quest & Design :ii:

WELL WELL

Astron Hues

d'moon books

Preface

So much in life is design,
designed as desired,
designed interior decor,
structures, sport rules,
and so on, so forth.

Design speeches?
Sure, as lots trained,
        for business
or talkings elsewhere.
Design sense?
Eh...

Design spacecrafts into space?
Surely, there are plenty.
Celestral Design of planets,
Milky Way, has been
a constant muse.

Fun to design,
Challenge to quest:
can life journey be designed?
How about destiny,
as all desire happiness?

Cosmos is gargantuan,
Earth solid, little known.
Lucky you, lucky me,
beings being here
to enjoy, to explore.

Join me!

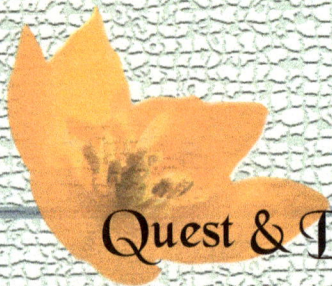

Quest & Design

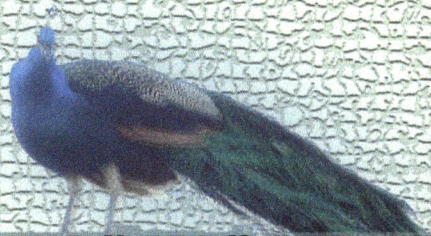

Well Well

Section i   16 - 39

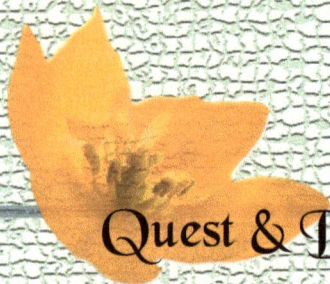

Quest & Design

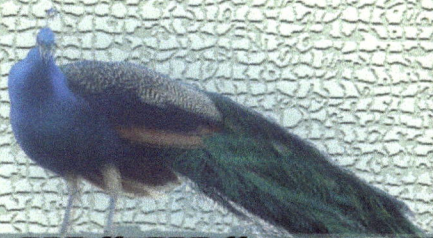

Well Well

Quest & Design

✦Four Steps Wiser✦
- Reading and Reflection Vol. 04
released in 2021 (in full color)

✦Five Steps Wiser✦
- Reading and Reflection Vol. 05
released in 2021
designed art b&w interior print

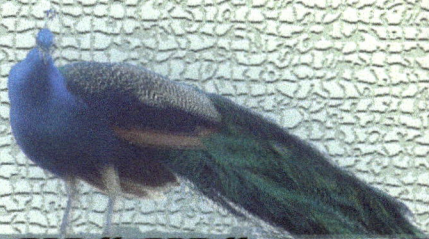

Well Well

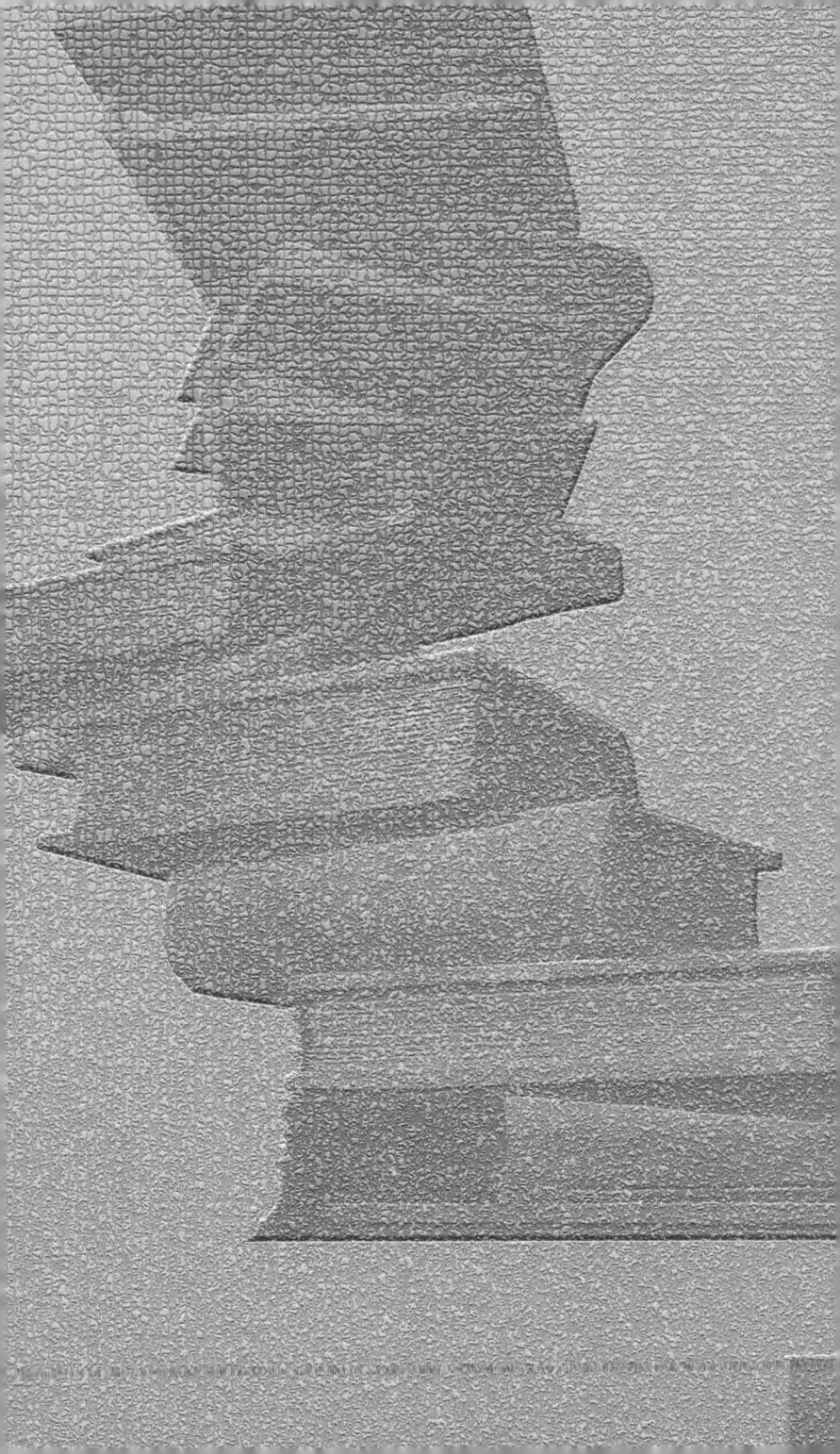

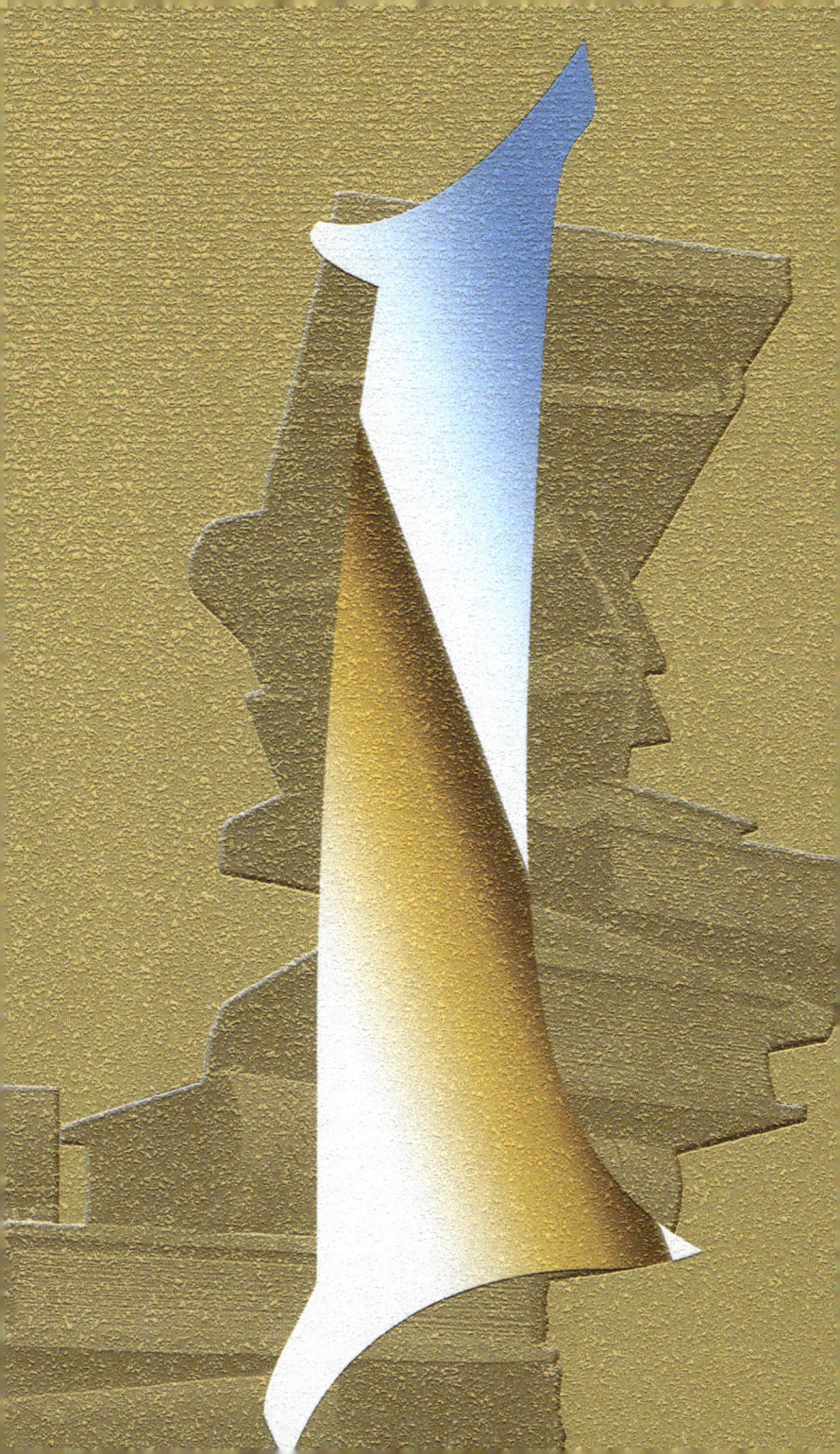

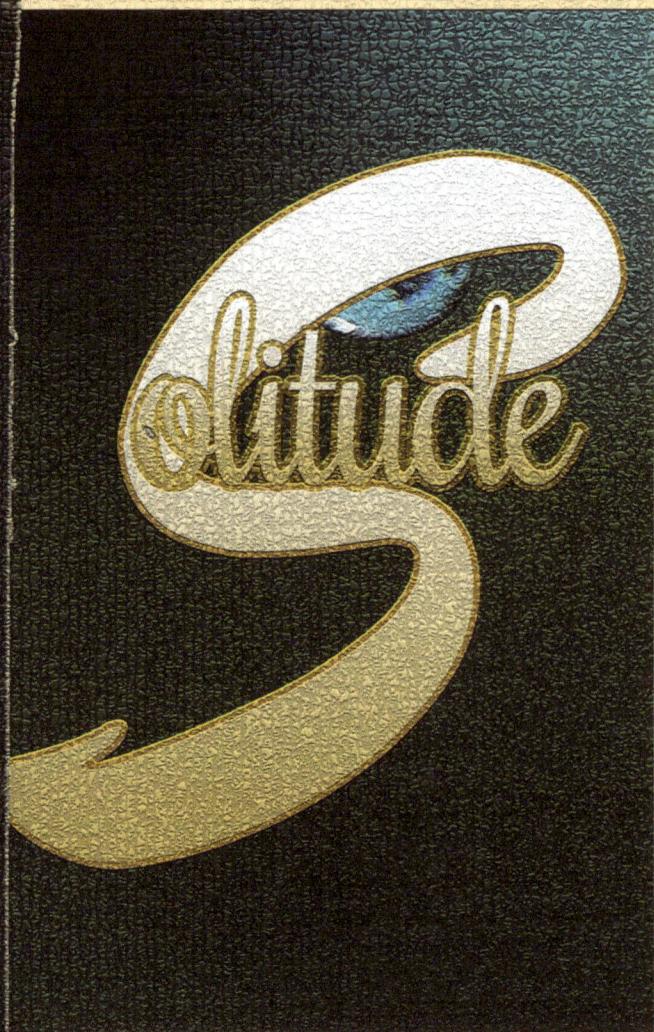

Well Well

1. Snow. Solitude.

Morning,
Snow, thoughtful, soundless,
melting upon my face.
Trees and houses, all in solitude.
Then, wind, storm.
Winter does as winter would
usually do. Piercing
cold takes folks by surprise.
Not wearing warm clothes?
We do as we usually do, turn
on whatever devices to heat up.

Convenience followed by
inconvenience:
Power surges plunge
thousands into darkness,
as it happened in previous winters.
Now, it happens again.

Nature offers us what we need
and perhaps teachings as well.

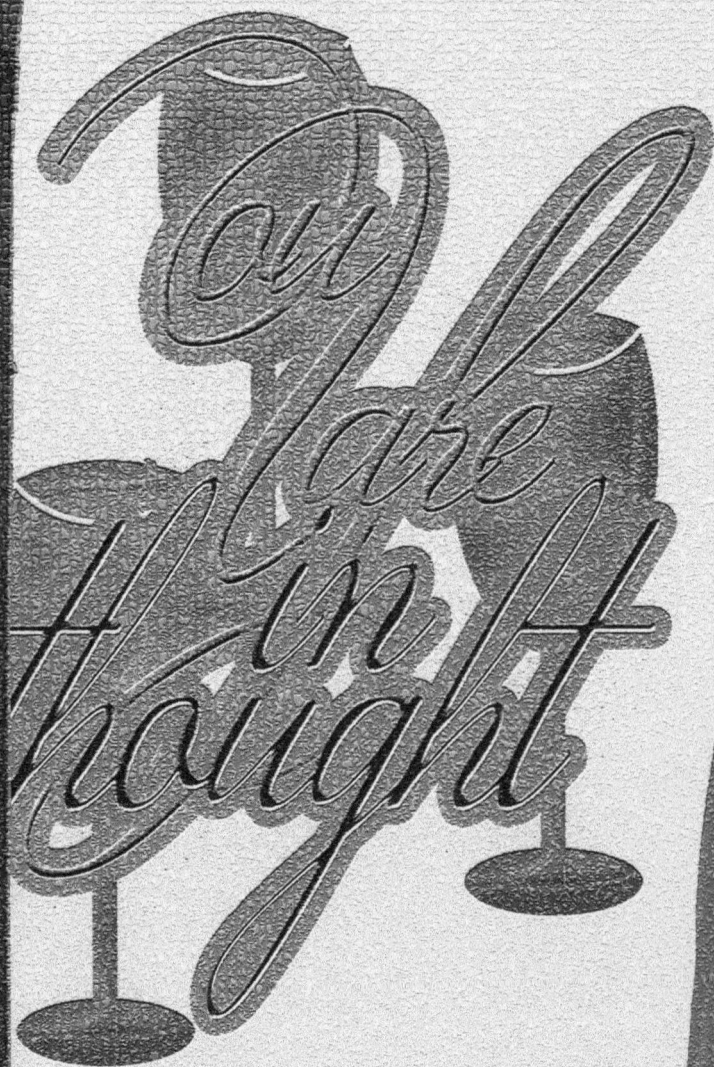

Our Lare in thought

Well Well

2. "Luxury", Lost

Guests inside, sitting around,
holding glasses of wine.
Cheese, snacks,
on solid wood coffee table. Talking,
sports game on big screen,
crackling fire flickering in fireplace...

What a relaxful time of leisure,
and as we would often do.
But no more:
the runaway facemasks still not
yet retreated back to hospitals.
Neither does caution:
dine out or eat in,
work in offices or remotely?
Switch back and forth.

Never thought, simple joys,
as we would often have, is now
"Luxury", and lost.

Quest & Design

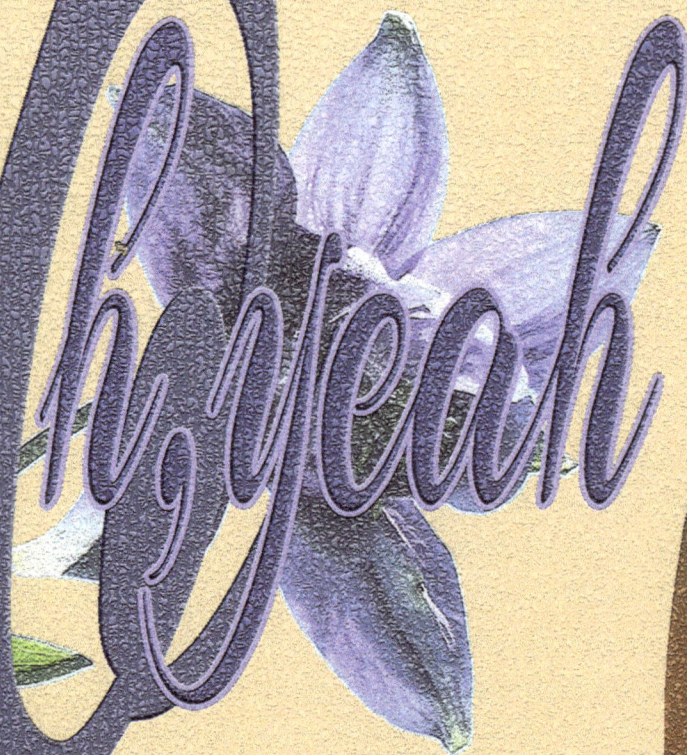

Well Well

3. Granted? No more.

Luxuries are still around
in luxury homes,
luxury offices, or luxury hotels,
such as furniture, souvenirs, collections
motionless without
party-goers' attention.
Unable to speak to one another,
their steward is alone, feeling lonely,
perhaps the luxury things
feel lonely too.

Luxury of luxuries is to meet
with dear friends in person,
or to chat with acquaintances
face to face at get-together.

Is that part of thousands
of years' civilization... So
accustomed, to take for granted?
No more.

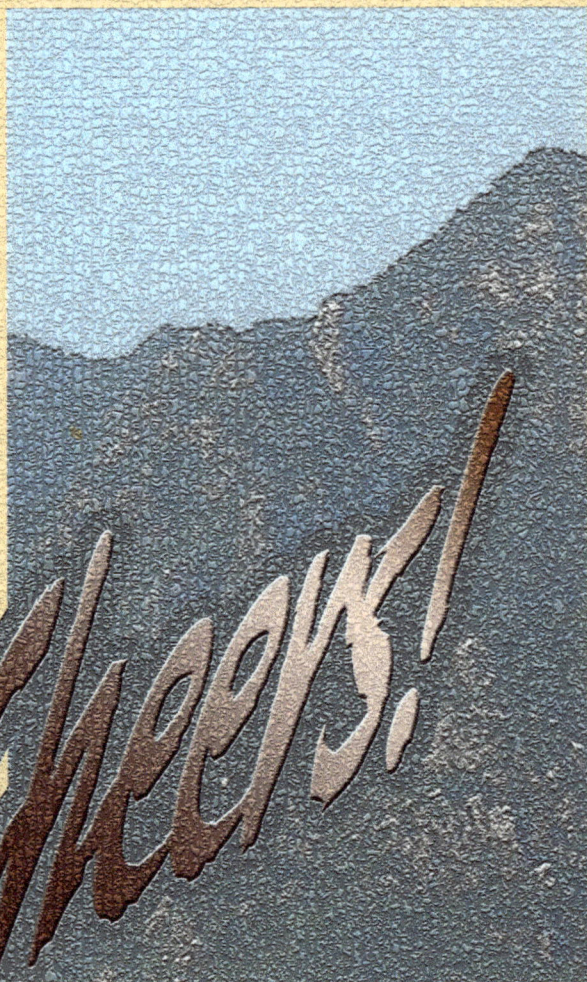

Well Well

4. Catch it when you can!

Things lost, things valued.
What else, not anymore
to be taken for granted?
The never-returning time –
youngest year of all is here,
and on the way leaving,
by day, by week, by month,
not nodding goodbye,
nor slowing down,
sliding away, passing by,
never coming back.

Catch the sunrise...
catch the sunlight...
catch the youthfulness...
Future in Fashion of Haste
catch it when we can!

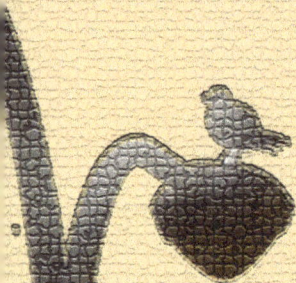

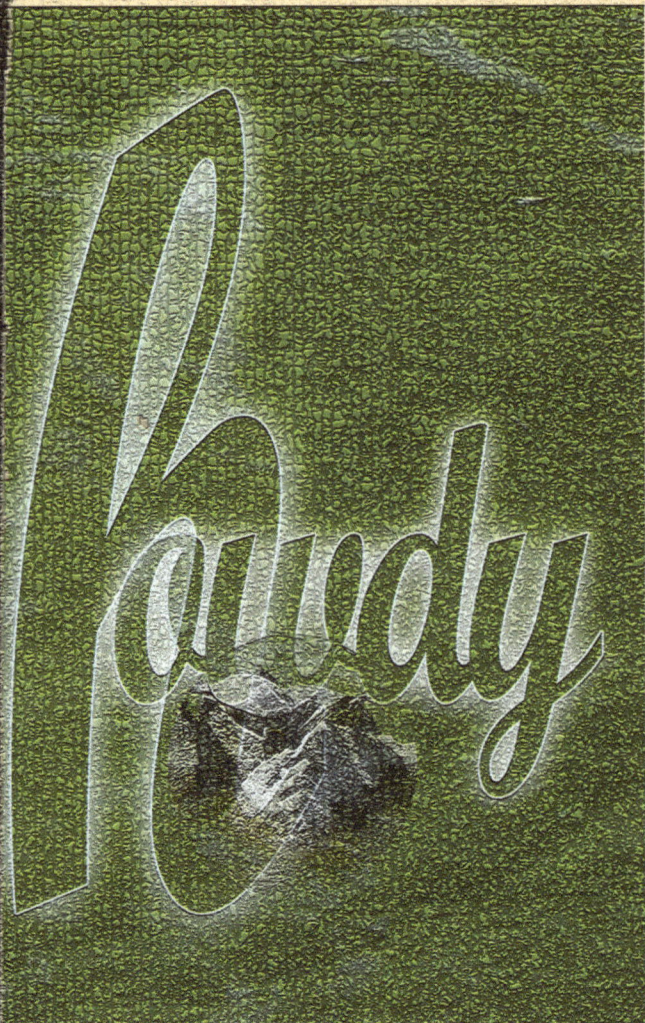

Well Well

5. Time is Life.

Indeed, on the constantly
vanishing time Life rides,
fading away as gentle as
shadow cast on the ground. Birthday
is celebrated year in year out,
until the day to bid farewell.
In between, when little, we
are impatient to grow up,
learning, having fun;
at teenage, throwing away
tons of time, hours, days...

Time aplenty, granted – there's
always tomorrow, next week,
next month, or next year.
Time always available,
offered without cost... until
someday words uttered:
"I'm old."
"Old?"
"Nonsense".

Well Well

6. Centenarians: You are young!

Yes, young as we are,
and much younger than
Centenarians
(over hundred thousands out there,
and the number
is still growig bigger).
How much time ahead?
No one can tell, no one knows.
We do enjoy time
when life is at ease,
not stretched, not stressed.
We love to walk or run
around with light steps,
heart filled with sunshine,
spot pleasant things
to smile about.

Centenarians are right:
we are young!

Quest & Design

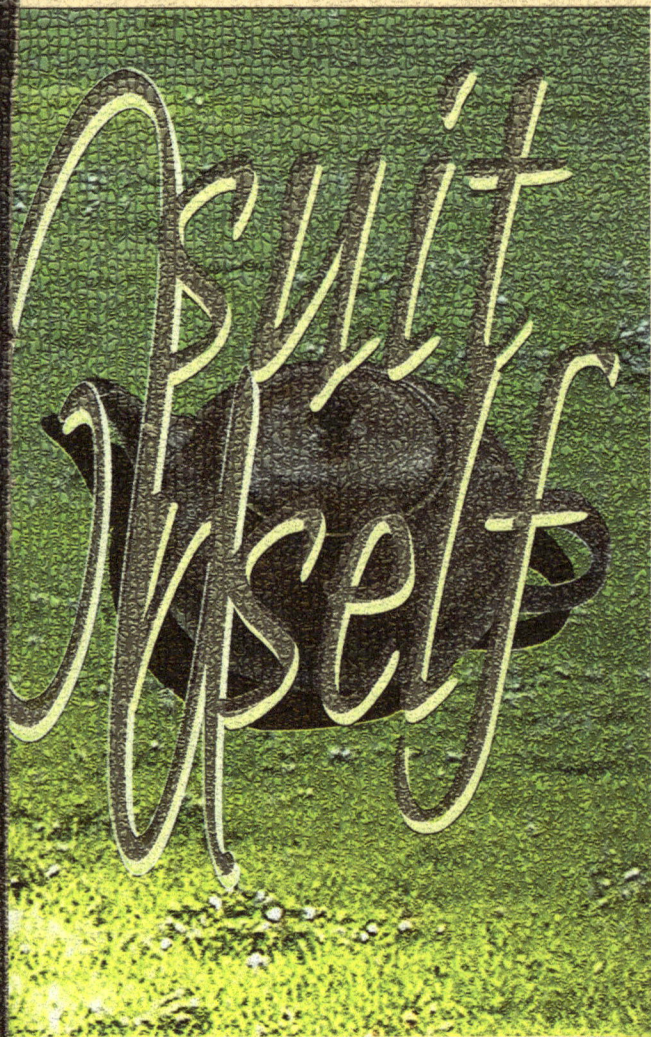

Well Well

7. Good time.
Life is good.

Where and when do we feel
we are having a good time –
when being self?
when smiling, giggling, laughing?
when scoring on sporting field?
when strolling along beach?
when bird-watching?
when visiting an art gallery?
when savoring favourite food?
when catching up on reading?...

Your list of a good time
might be much longer.
Good times, plenty, certainly
compose a good life,
desired by all.

Time
is Life

Well Well

8. "Treasure": unwasted time

Reality offers no exception –
24 hours per day, 365 days a year.
No more, no less.
Working hours are long.
Sleeping hours cannot be reduced.
To-do list hardly gets shorter.
Weekends and vacations disappear fast.

Extra hours for a good time.
Dig from bundles
of huddled mess, sitting in
corners, or shuffled away
at bottom of bookshelves.
A bundle of huddled mess,
mounting stress.

Turning pressure away,
no time to waste,
extra time for more good times –
Treasure to be discovered.

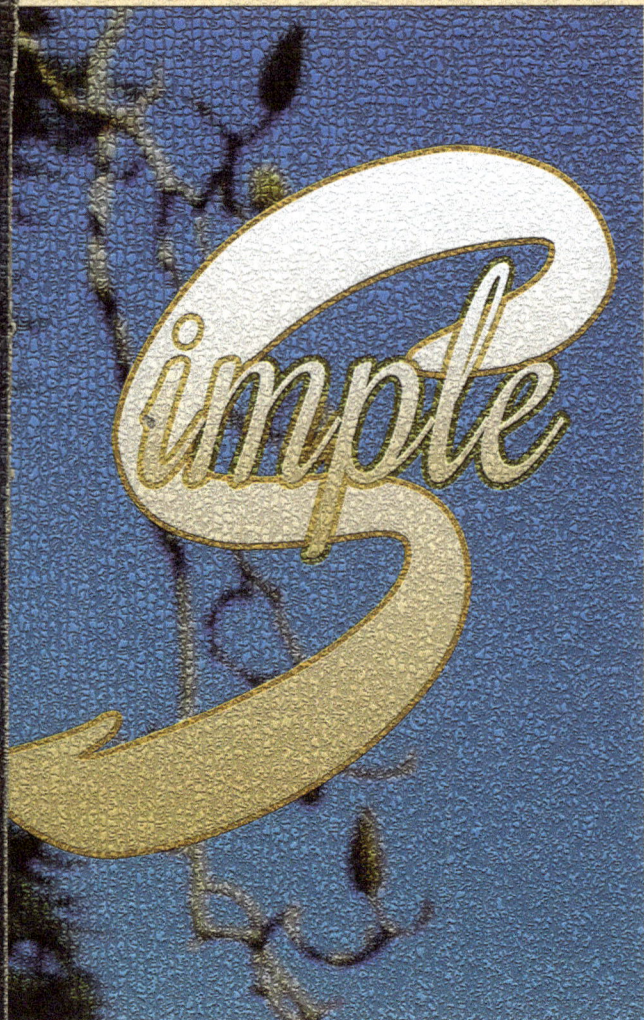

Well Well

9. Simplicity delivers more.

Looking up into sky, blue,
looking around, snow, white.
Gigantic vast. Simple.
We, souls, far littler, and
how simpler are we –
when talking about goals,
multiple;
when talking about tasks,
multiple;
when talking about devices,
multiple. However,
simplest designed programs are
loved most...

Similarly, simple procedure,
simple process, rewarding:
fewer errors,
more efficiency;
less overwork,
more time to sip beer.

Quest & Design

Good
g'day

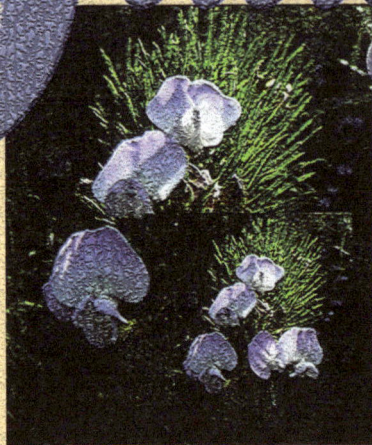

Well Well

10. Well well, bargain with self.

Simplicity delivers focus,
precision,
releases us from anxiety to have
more good time –
    brief to-do list,
    straighten out the complicated,
    reduce redundancy,
    avoid unnecessary repetition,
    single out significant goals
if too many.

Simplicity delivers
    sense of accomplishment
    easiness, bon appetit, sweet sleep.
Simplicity delivers more good time
    which ripples far,
    far beyond.

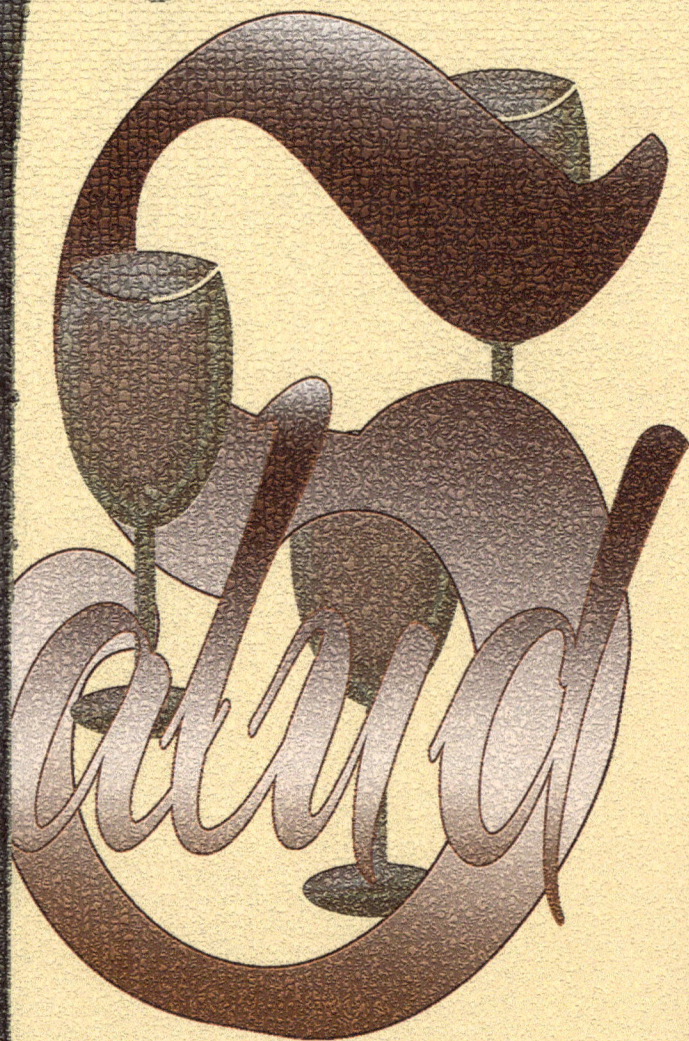

Well Well

11. In Thought

Good time, plenty.
Life is good.
Treasure, unwasted time
is waiting to be discovered –
having plenty of good time is
desirable, tempting, irresistable.

Free will is challenged:
well well, have to bargain with self,
        just as a dollar saved,
            a dollar earned;
        time unwasted,
            treasure discovered.

Carry good time, joyful smile,
        and Fortune of Health,
march into merrier tommorow.
Life is good!

Dear friends,
you are all in thought!

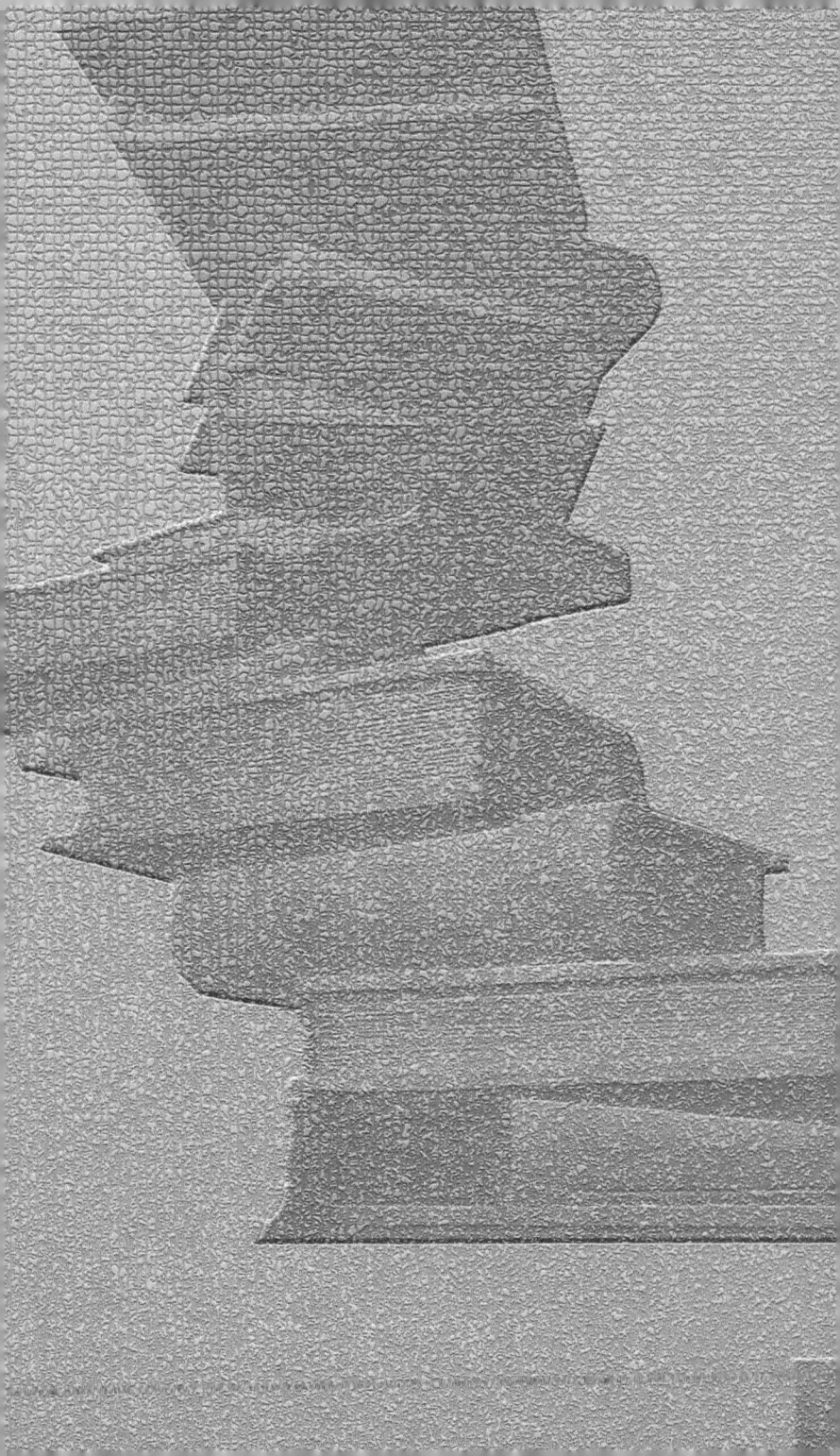

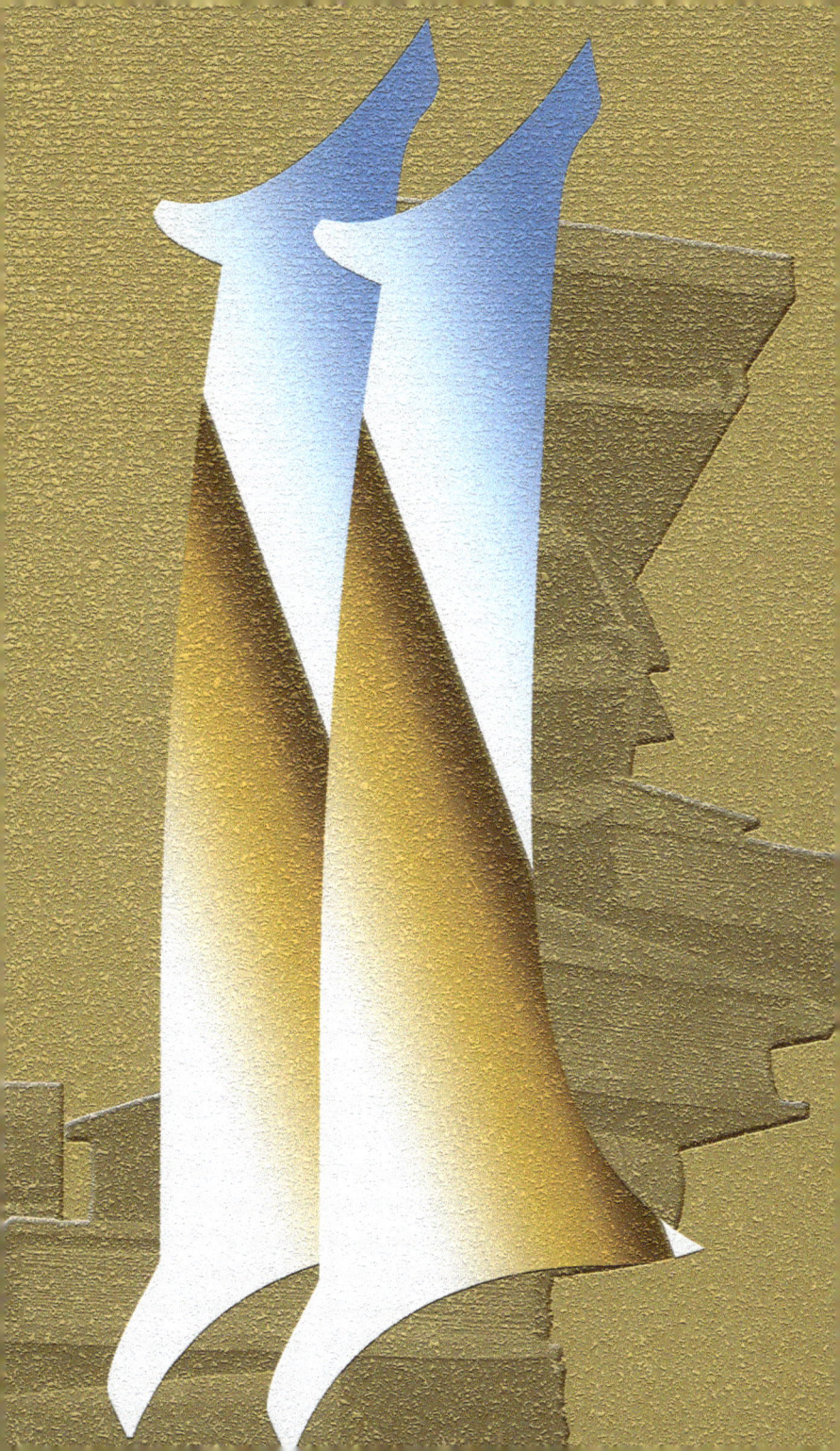

Race of the Century

Well Well

It is the race of the century.
Yes! 40 million audience
to hear the call.
It is a race of destiny
between a horse from
the west coast; and a horse
from the east coast.
It is a match race.
Match race? Unlikely matched.

15 hands vs 18 hands high.
The numbers of size spell out
an unlikely match.
Who would think otherwise?
Might be doomed by his name of
small crackers,
seabiscuit was too small
to impress.

Quest & Design

40 million
hear the call
businesses closed
half day

44

Well Well

Unlikely match. Indeed.
In addition to being little,
Seabiscuit indulges in long hours
of eating and sleeping, lulling
under a tree.
Lazy as he is, yet not spared
as a racehorse
he is, a hopeless loser,
heavily scheduled for races
to boost other horses' confidence.
Seabiscuit is sired by Hard Tack
(grandfather Man o'War).
Fortunate.
Also unfortunate.

Quest & Design

Nov 1st 1938 –
Pimlico
17000 gallons
of lemonade
2000 kegs
of beer
60000
hot dogs

Well Well

Unlikely match,
per market value,
price on champion War Admiral
at least 5 digits.
Seabiscuit? Sold at $2,000,
the little horse sleeps
a lot and eats a lot,
often beaten up
"running in circles",
consequently, bitter,
and very hot-tempered.

Match race unlikely

Well Well

Having lost more than
his unimpressive wins,
and with an imperfect knee,
Seabiscuit is to challenge
War Admiral
of perfect form, perfect record.
Any factors
in favor of Seabiscuit?
If nothing is overlooked,
then his chance to win is slim,
as the scale entirely leans
to one side.

Unlikely match.

Quest & Design

15 hands
high vs
18 hands

Well Well

Match race?
Seabiscuit is said
("to run out on some cow track"
while War Admiral is a
champion horse,
Triple Crown winner.

Match race, regardless how
unlikely, is on.
As required by
War Admiral's terms,
over a distance of 1 and 3/16th
miles (9 and 1/2 furlongs)
held at War Admiral's home
track, Pimlico, Baltimore.
Start with a bell, but,
without usual starting gate.

Quest & Design

Seabiscuit vs War Admiral

Well Well

Pimlico, Baltimore,
November 1 1938.
At 10 in the morning,
parking space is only available
15 blocks away.
Thousands of gallons of
lemonade, beer,
Thousands of hot dogs
are prepared...
Businesses closed,
allowing employees
a half day off to hear the call.
Beside the radio,
on the trees, infields,
crowds are everywhere.

Quest & Design

War Admiral

Triple Crown

champion

54

Well Well

Breathtaking moment.
At the starting line,
the match race of the century.
No gate to divide two impatient,
agitated racehorses,
eager to kick off.
18-hand tall War Admiral
is so sure to win.
Anyone there to lift up
the 15-hand one's confidence?
Certainly not.
Seabiscuit seems not at all
intimidated by the big
Triple Crown winner,
intimidating.

Seabiscuit

sold at

$2000

Well Well

The confidence in himself
must touch the sky.
He takes the lead, by one length,
by two lengths.
At the back stretch,
he is held back,
waits for his rival,
until head to head,
shoulder to shoulder,
and eye to eye.
A brief courtesy greeting
like an athlete,
Seabiscuit is saying hello
to his competitor,
"hey buddy, take it easy,
I'll take the prize, see ya."

3.25 miles
War Admiral's
home track

Well Well

And in a split second,
with free will taking destiny
into his own speed,
Seabiscuit dashes out, gallops.
"Seabiscuit by one length,
leading War Admiral",
"Seabiscuit by two lengths,
War Admiral fading away",
"Seabiscuit by three and half
lengths"...
flying past the finish line.

Unlikely winner
at unlikely matched match race.

Quest & Design

|-to-|
start with bell
no gate

Well Well

Back then,
40 million heard the call.
The award-winning movie
Seabiscuit
(owner Charles Howard
played by Jeff Bridges,
trainer Tom Smith
by Chris Cooper,
daily jockey Red Pollard
by Tobey Maguire,
match race jockey George Woolf
by Gary Stevens)
brings back the race of century,
over decades of time.
Hundreds of millions
would hear the call.

Quest & Design

Would you
bet on
winner by
3.5 lengths?

Well Well

A superior horse to be spotted
is desired.
Training to be a champion
is designed.
The win is not in the legs
but "in the heart",
as it happened which is far,
far beyond the desired design,
isn't it?

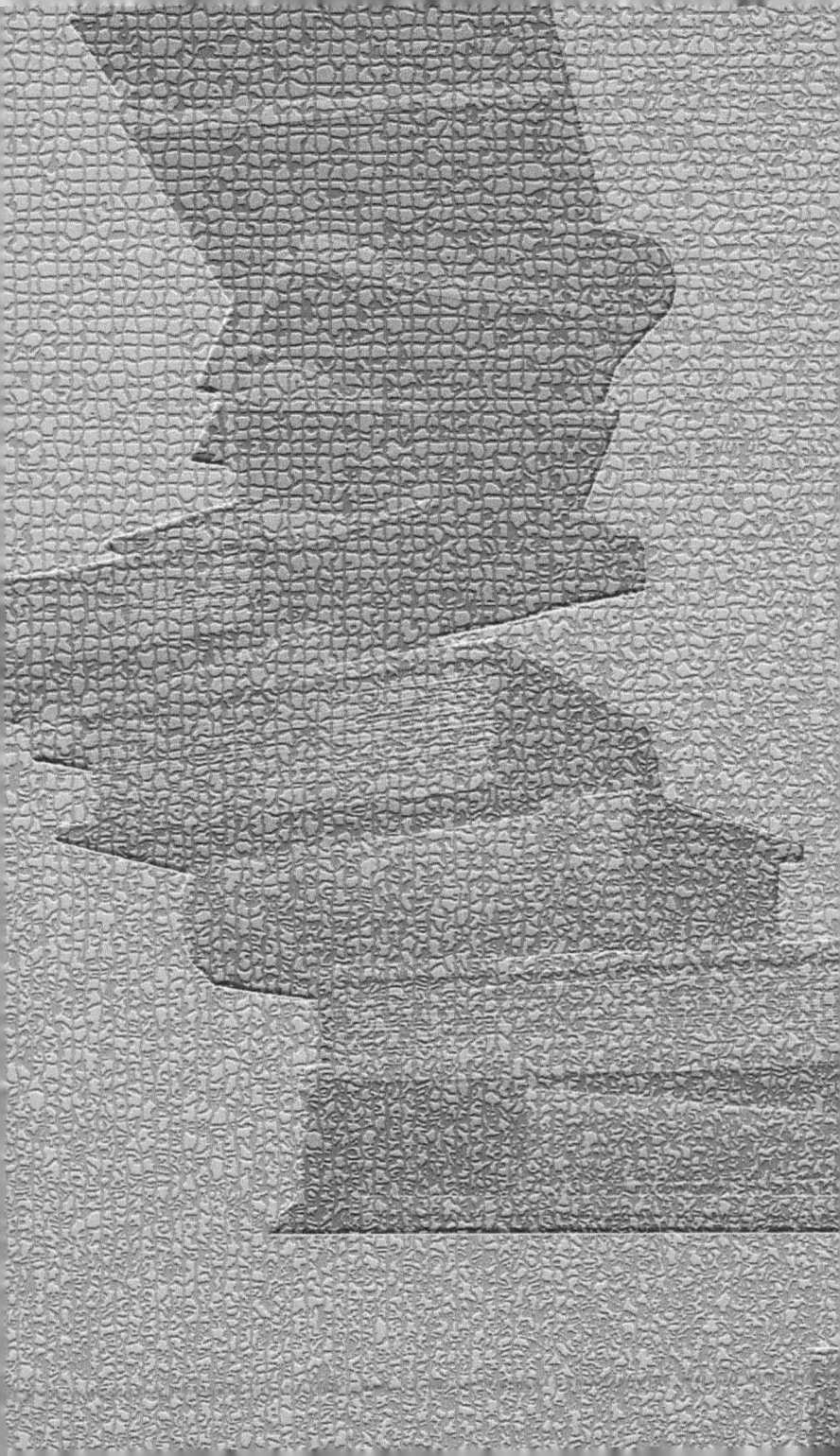

Appendix A

Read more

Appendix

Xoom books

FourStepsWiser

Dear Goodluck

World
Culture
Pictorial
Reading &
Reflection
Vol. 4

Read more

Xtreme Books

Five Steps Wiser

Dear Goodluck

World
Culture
Pictorial
Reading &
Reflection
Vol 5

Appendix

L

D.Moore
Book of L

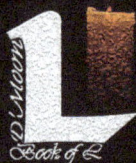

ISBN 978-1-933187-94-5

90000

9 781933 187945

Read more

BOOK OF L²

Quotable Wit & Wisdom

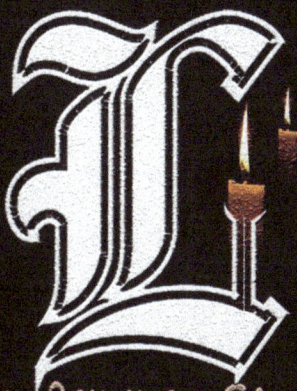

L

Dr. Common Sense

dmoon books

Appendix

Love speaks for Romance,

Read More

*Love speaks
more for
Compassion.*

- Luffeed

Appendix

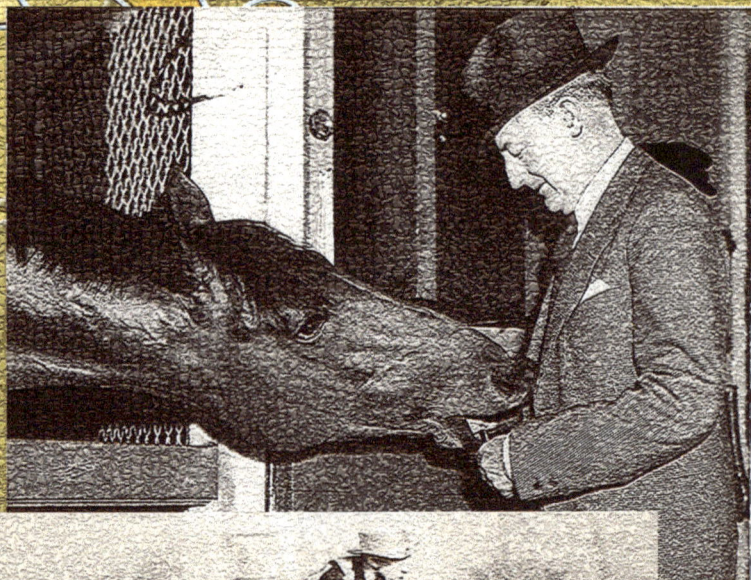

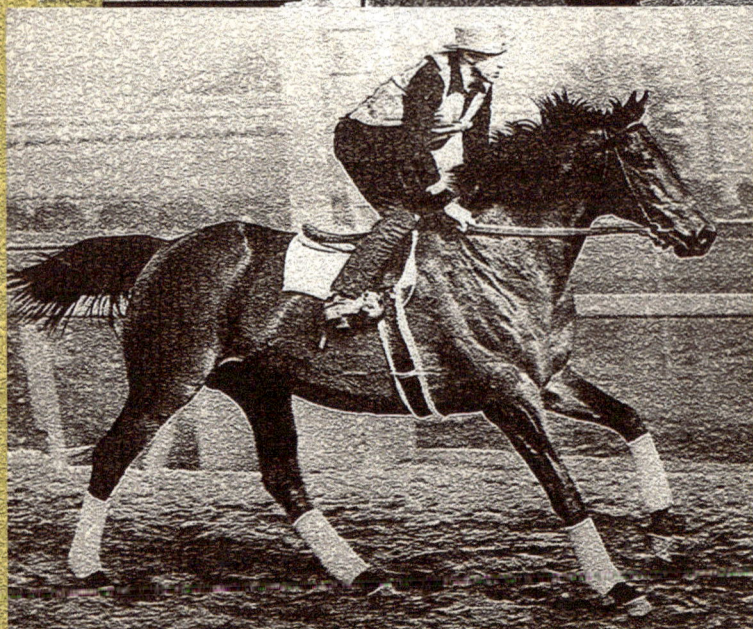

Read more

Seabiscuit's team in life –
owner (L)
Charles Howard
trainer (R)
Tom Smith
daily jockey (R)
Red Pollard
match race jockey (L)
George Woolfe

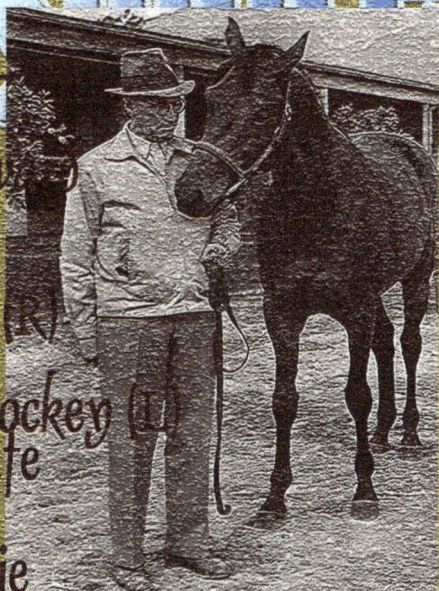

stars in movie
"Seabiscuit" –
owner:
Jeff Bridges
trainer:
Chris Cooper
jockey:
Tobey Maguire
George Woolf:
Gary Stevens
image credit
Seabiscuit
Heritage
Foundation

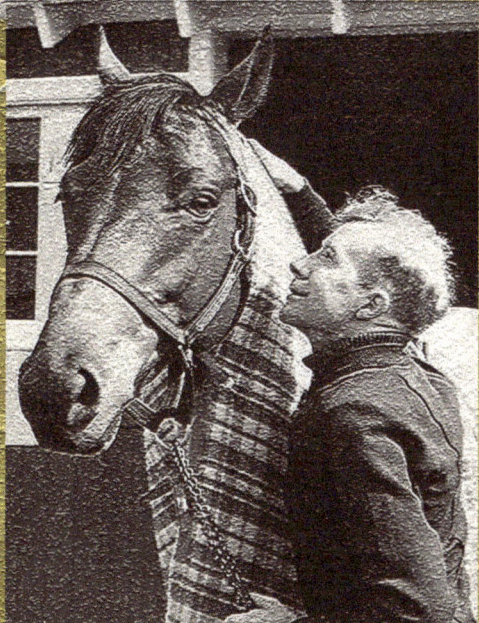

.

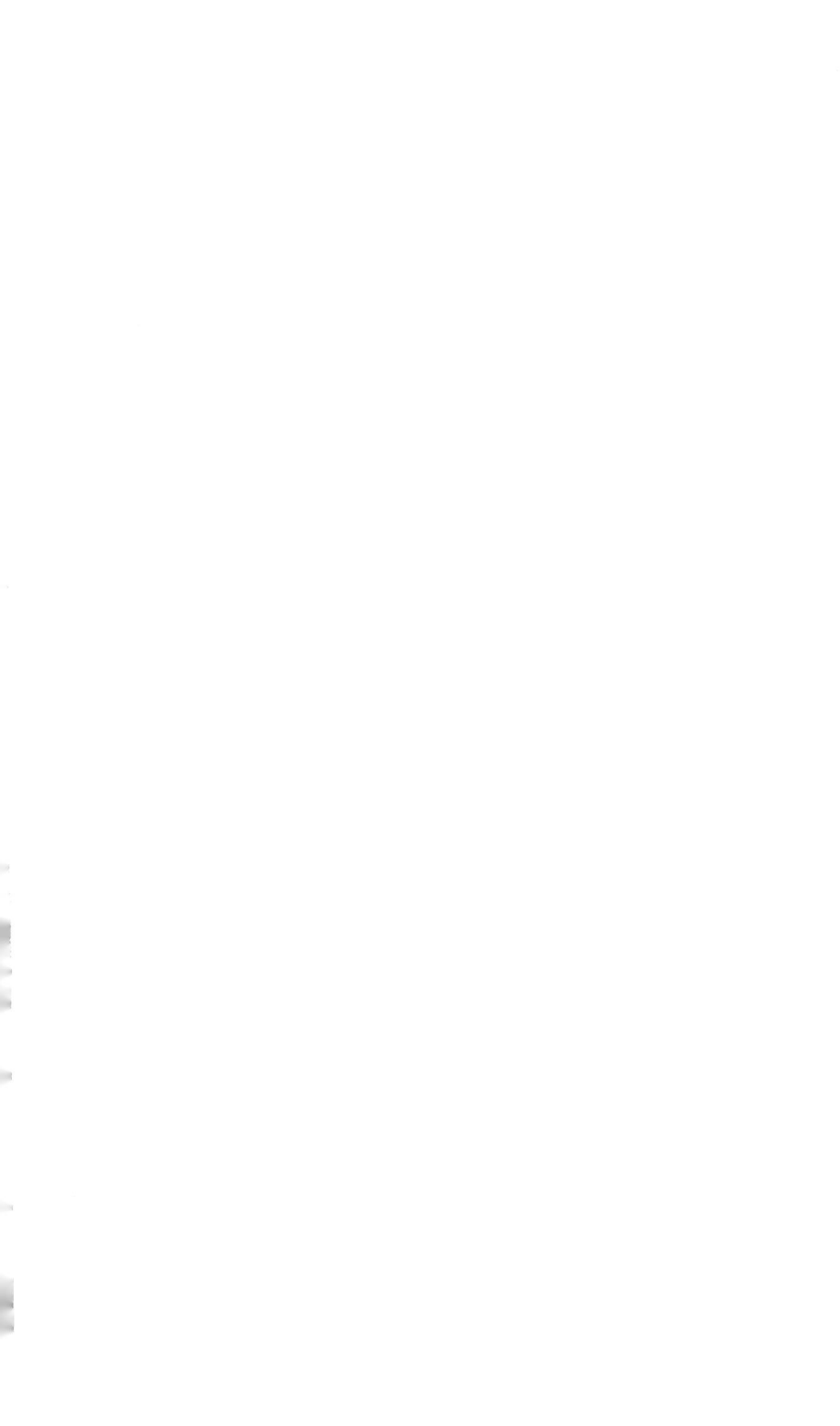